You Got This Consulting

Self Esteem/Self Confidence Inventory & Proliferation Program

By

Israel-Shannon M. Saunders

For: Michael Allen,

Thank you for teaching me about hope

This presentation is published by I. Saunders Ink.

604-B Gomains Avenue

Chapel Hill, North Carolina 27516

brothersaunders@aol.com

<u>Please send any and all correspondence, donations, requests for speaking engagements to the above street address with the name Israel-Shannon Saunders as the recipient.</u>

<u>Donations will assist the Orange County Sickle Cell Support Group</u>

Table of Contents

Welcome/Greeting

I would like to welcome each of you to the You Got This Consulting Self Esteem and Self Confidence Inventory and Proliferation Program.

It is a long name, but what it means is this…

WHEN IT COMES TO DISCOVERING AND BUILDING SELF CONFIDENCE-YOU GOT THIS!!!!

It is my sincere belief and mission to inform each of you that there is no obstacle in your personal or professional life that can withstand the power that you hold at all times to heap encouragement upon yourself. So I welcome you into the journey of a lifetime that I hope you will hold onto even in your deepest moments of pain, frustration, and despair. I wrote this program for all of you here today because I certainly know that You Got This!

Welcome all and let's get started.

Purpose, Goals, and Aims of YGTC

Someone may ask or be wondering what exactly the purpose of You Got This Consulting is and what all of these exercises and surveys are even about.

Doesn't it appear obvious that the time that a sickle cell patient or a sickle cell family member or a trusted advocate who is that neighbor or the rest of the truly uneducated or undereducated world is greatly limited by the eccentric schedule sickle cell diseases follow?

Excuse me sir, but don't you realize that sickle cell is said to me to be permanent, life altering, and relentless?

My answer to these questions is a resounding YES!!

YES…I do know that a sickle cell patient, family member, neighbor/community, and the rest of the world are on incredibly tight schedules due to sickle cell's reach into lives.

YES…I do know that sickle cell is said to be a permanent heavyweight match between yourselves and its presence. And that is exactly why this program to en-courage you was developed.

The purpose of this program is to empower each of you to reach beyond whatever has been said about the fruitfulness of your lives and learn to speak words of life and comfort and hope over yourselves.

The goal of this effort is to encourage each of you to develop your God given muscles to speak life over yourself. Some call this faith while others call it positive self talk. In either case, the words you say to yourself should always reflect your ability to succeed beyond your current position. We will exercise and strengthen this positive self talk muscle through this work…that I can guarantee.

The aims of this work are to produce in each of you the library of positive thinking, speaking, and acting that you might gain a brighter view of life whether it rains, sleets, hails, snows, tsunamis, earthquakes, or whatever other weather event you can think of arrives. My chief aim is for you to realize the strength that you always have with you to determine your path forward.

Are you ready to make your darkest thoughts rumble?

A Bit of My Story

I was born November 27. It was Thanksgiving Day. She always reminds me on my birthday that it was 8:08am when I entered the world.

6 months later my family learned that I had sickle cell disease…whatever that was. Older generations had dealt with it, yet a definitive name hardly ever stuck. Some

called it arthritis, others the biting disease. In 1981, 6 months after I arrived it was called sickle cell disease.

I can't recall the time from 6 months of age to about 5 years very clearly besides the numerous hospital visits. At 5 years old, I became more aware of my mom, dad, and then sister. I used to dislike her presence so much.

My life would never be the same. Several things happened at 5 years old for me. At 5 years, I started school. The school buses looked like hungry yellow bananas that swallowed up kids and took them away from mommy and daddy and sent them to a land of carpets and kickball and math. Those were the best ways I could describe the school buses and the schools we were taken to.

At 5, my dad was apart from the family for a while, and so my mom became the most important person in my life. To this day I do not know how she made it all work out. Between her job, my illness, the hospitals, an unfolding sickle cell disease reality, our family challenges, and the crazy weather where we lived then, she held our little family together for the next 9 years.

At 10 years old, I had a stroke. It was very alarming coming out of that familiar convenience store en route to grandma's and falling down to my knees unable to get them to do what they had always done.

It was very disappointing because going to grandma's meant a few pieces of fried chicken, maybe some turnips, stuffing, mashed potatoes, whew, got a little carried away. But grandma's always meant her fried chicken for me. I would not get to have that planned meeting with her fried chicken that day because the call to UNC changed those plans. The doctors just kept telling my mother that I couldn't have had a stroke, but the symptoms were all there in front of us.

So, at 10 years old I was a stroke victim and that meant a new treatment called the blood transfusion. The treatment was to keep fresh blood flowing in my system to hopefully prevent any other stroke(s) and complications.

It was a time of great uncertainty. Taking blood transfusion therapy meant a couple of things. First, it meant a 45 minute drive from Roxboro to Chapel Hill two times a month. All of us in this room know, however, that you can't set a watch by sickle cell's consistency.

The trips to Chapel Hill became more frequent because the regional hospital in Person County was inadequately staffed, stocked, and structured when handling sickle cell crisis. We learned the hard way.

Not long after the blood transfusions, we discovered a new complication. Having so many blood transfusions caused too much iron to stay in my blood. The treatment for this was chelation therapy. Every night mama had to stick a needle into my chest to lower the iron levels. I was too active in the daytime with school and other activities to do chelation during the day. The medicine needed eight hours to filter through.

Chelation therapy soon became troublesome and a new idea was needed to treat my illness. A new treatment was suggested that would take all of my bone marrow out, put new bone marrow in, and watch for the new life expected beyond sickle cell disease. A bone marrow transplant would remove my body's blueprint to make sickle cells because the body's cells are all made in the bone marrow.

My family members were checked to see whose bone marrow matched my own. The perfect candidate arrived. It was she who I loathed her existence when she was newly born. My sister was chosen. She was 8 years old and I was 13. They (the doctors) asked if we wanted to try and we said yes.

March 1, 1994 was the big day. I had chemotherapy to remove all the sickle cell from my body. I was given a special room that filtered the air differently from the rest of the hospital rooms on a special wing with special staff because of this truly special opportunity.

The bone marrow arrived later that morning in a bag that looked very much like a bag of blood used for blood transfusions. It dripped in very slowly. Finally, it was complete. Now began the 100 day wait to see if my body rejected the new bone marrow from my sister. The rejection is called graft-versus-host disease. Then the 100 days were over. I could go home for good. It was time to start a new life.

It was strange at first to hear Dr. Wiley say that a successful treatment could end my need for doctor's visits completely. That was a long reach from where I was at then. All I knew or could see was sickle cell.

I have gone back to the hospital several times since 1994 but not one time has been for the treatment of sickle cell disease. That part of my life that seemed so permanent has eroded from my view.

On March 1, 2013, I celebrated 19 years without sickle cell disease. I share a bit of my story with you not to isolate you from myself or to present you or I as vastly different from one another, but to give you hope that the darkest moments must open and yield some sunshine. I am not certain exactly how or what form your sunshine shall take, but I do firmly believe that it is on its way into your life.

Why Self Confidence Is Important To Us Here?

Self confidence is important to us here in this setting and in this time because it offers a doorway to reach success. If you are able to see that you can build a muscle in your arm by lifting a 5 pound weight, then you should have no trouble seeing the same technique in building your self confidence. I encourage you to lift your positive outlook and words to exercise your confidence level.

You Can Do This Alone or In A Group

Self confidence is reachable whether you are in alone or in a crowd. It may seem like you are unable to bring self confidence to your situation when you are without any companionship. I would say that this is the best time to exercise your technique. You can create ways to tell and remind yourself that you are worth the effort. This also works when you are in a group setting. You can lift your own self confidence by giving positive words and feedback to those around of you. In the workplace, this is known as **emotional intelligence**. When you take the time to tell yourself or to remind others that they are worth it, that you are valuable, important, and necessary, the day's worries clear up a little bit. You have to give yourself doses of encouragement in those places where your rough times are biggest. Let your encouragement outperform your toughest places.

The Definitions

Goal Setting- written plan one reviews showing desired goals and their expected completion times

Virtue- the goodness and rightness of your actions

Positive self talk/outlook- language used to encourage and give a positive view to yourself

Self efficacy- viewing ourselves mastering skills alongside others with similar KSA's as ourselves

KSA's- knowledge, skills, and abilities

Self Confidence- the ability to consider purpose and find peace with life's journey

Goals- specific target to accomplish in the future

Self esteem- the general outlook that we can deal with life's circumstances

Competence- platform where self confidence is built

Emotional Intelligence- the attitude taken to solve problems in person to person interaction(s)

Let's Look At The Tools

There are several tools I have found useful in this course: I will share them with you, but the greatest satisfaction can only find you as you insert and invest yourself into the process given here. The tools for this effort are worksheets that look at where self confidence can be used, 6, 12, and 10 year individual goal lists, list of people who can encourage us to meet our goals, list of positive self talk affirmations and goal mapping charts.

Where This Works

The concept of believing in yourself and in your abilities to function effectively, to show yourself as valuable and important, is wrapped up in your readiness to monitor your self confidence. There is no place where you cannot practice building your self concept, your self image up, so that you can manage even the toughest situations.

This course gives you a formula for focusing on loving you and caring for you. You are not excluded from the ability to build your own self confidence and the benefit may be greater for you than for some others because of where you have been. My goal is to help you to focus on being a better you for you first and then for everyone else. You live in a community, but if you cannot motivate and inspire and love yourself through good words and living then the work ahead of you is a bit tougher.

I am showing this formula because I have found myself doing these very things over and over again when I faced my tough situations. Every day is not going to be the easiest to face...which we all know in this room. But as we hear about the importance of IEP's, awareness, building positive relationships, and having some anchor in the rough storms of sickle cell disease, we can become greater for the effort of organizing ourselves and exercising our self confidence muscles.

Goals, Goal Mapping, & Vision Boarding

You have the ability to set goals. Setting goals helps build your self confidence by giving you the focus and the determination to complete the goal. As one goal is met or in progress other goals can be in the process also. One important thing is that goals must be written down to show record of the process for yourself and for others. A very valuable tool that is similar is the resume. Resumes record the efforts you have made in volunteer and paid work, the education you have gathered and the goal that you are reaching for in the future. We present this because each of these areas offers you visual proof of your goal and your progress.

Above all, my friends, remember that You Got This!

Enjoy the journey and the achieving,

Pastor Israel-Shannon Saunders

Activity 1- Where Can I Use Self Confidence?

See if you can find the occupation of each example.

1. I hear hundreds of children a week screaming as I drive a _____ to carry them to a day's new learning experience. Self confidence is vital.

2. The _____ has lots of quiet time while some people bow their heads and pray.

3. I give out judgments and recommendations for persons who have committed crimes at the _____. This takes incredible self confidence.

4. When I am on the _____ I have to have a lot of self confidence to rush into the water if I need to help someone breathe again.

5. My job at the _____ requires a lot of self confidence as I try to see how their heart will work better.

Activity 2- Make It Plain

Write down 2 short term, 2 medium term and 2 long term goals. Short term = now - 6 months, medium term = 6 months – 1 year, long term = 1 year – 10 years.

In the next 6 months, I would like to accomplish these 2 things in my life:

    (1) I would like to <u>get a library card.</u> {example}

    (2) I would like to _____.

    (3) I would like to _____.

In the next 1 year, I would like to accomplish these 4 things in my life:

    (1) I would like to <u>begin writing an autobiography.</u> {example}

    (2) I would like to _____.

    (3) I would like to _____.

In the next 10 years, I would like to accomplish these 4 things in my life:

    (1) I would like to <u>save $20,000 dollars.</u> {example}

    (2) I would like to_____.

    (3) I would like to _____.

Activity 3- Accountability

Build a list of people who you can trust to boost your self confidence. List 4 people here.

1. I can trust _____ to boost my self confidence.

2. I can trust _____ to boost my self confidence.

3. I can trust _____ to boost my self confidence.

4. I can trust _____ to boost my self confidence.

Now where can you find these 4 people:

1. I can find someone to increase my self confidence in/at/ the _____.

2. I can find someone to increase my self confidence in/at/ the _____.

3. I can find someone to increase my self confidence in/at/ the _____.

4. I can find someone to increase my self confidence in/at/ the _____.

Activity 4 - Positive Self Talk

When times get tough we can call ourselves something positive. Below let's list a few of these positive statements to look to for strength when we face challenge.

1. When times are tough for me, I will close my eyes, take a deep breath, and say to myself
   _____.

2. When times are tough for me, I will close my eyes, take a deep breath, and say to myself
   _____.

3. When times are tough for me, I will close my eyes, take a deep breath, and say to myself
   _____.

4. When times are tough for me, I will close my eyes, take a deep breath, and say to myself
   _____.

5. When times are tough for me, I will close my eyes, take a deep breath, and say to myself
   _____.

6. When times are tough for me, I will close my eyes, take a deep breath, and say to myself
   _____.

<u>20 Positive Things To Say To Yourself In Challenge</u>

1. I am worth it!
2. I am able!
3. I can make it!
4. I am important!
5. I am better than this!
6. I can achieve my goals!
7. I am smart!
8. I matter!
9. I will not give up on myself!
10. I am giving!
11. I am a contributor!
12. I am willing to love!
13. I am able to succeed!
14. I am getting better!
15. I will accept the lesson!
16. I _____.
17. I _____.
18. I _____.
19. I _____.
20. I _____.

Note- Use these as you look in the mirror to gain strength or as you do Activity # 4.

Activity 5- Scenario Collection

The scenarios here intend to allow you to measure your internal tolls that play out in external ways. Each scenario has a few questions following to show the self awareness and community awareness functions of self confidence.

Scenario 1-

Samuel walks to the store with his dad every afternoon after he gets home from school. Samuel loves his dad very much and wants to show him in any way that he can. Samuel's dad says that Samuel is his reason to live and get himself together. Samuel doesn't know what to say to his dad, but just smiles and walks along. Samuel has been having trouble in class because he is not completing his homework. Samuel tells his teacher that he cannot concentrate at home.

1. What can Samuel do to let his dad know that he loves him?

2. What are some things that you can think of that can cause Samuel to complete his homework?

3. Are there any ways that Samuel's dad can help Samuel prepare for his success in school?

Scenario 2-

Diamond and Princess were the happiest sisters in the world. They did everything together: shopping, eating, studying, and reading to children at the elementary school. Diamond liked shopping for frog buttons, pens, and clothing, eating salads with lots of spinach and bulgur wheat, and studying the tropical rainforests. Princess liked shopping for state flags, globes, and law books, eating hummus and turkey sandwiches, and studying history and economics. One day the news reported that their uncle and their daddy were put in jail for pushing and hitting a middle school principal. Diamond asked Princess why she did not stay at home when their uncle and daddy were wanted to stay at home when their uncle and their daddy had a story to the incident and needed the family to support their rights.

1. Why do you think Diamond felt that her sister Princess was the person who made her the happiest in the world?

2. How do you know that people appreciate you?

3. Why do you think Diamond resisted her sister Princess' suggestion that she consider her position regarding their uncle and daddy's situation?

4. What do you think the reason could be that Princess resisted Diamond's suggestion that she consider the support of their uncle and daddy's situation a strain upon the family?

Scenario 3-

Damion lives in a community where the houses are unpainted, crumbling, and cannot provide enough space for all of the family members who live there. In Damion's house on Juniper Avenue lived Damion, his mother, his grandmother, grandfather, two uncles, aunt, four brothers and three sisters. They all shared 4 bedrooms. Damion's best friends were Hector and Simeon. Hector lived in a house on Drack Road with his father, his mother, and his two sisters. Everyone had their own bedroom. Simeon lived in a house on Halliwell Street that looked like a castle with his father, stepmother, uncle, and brother.

1. What is the major difference between Damion and two best his friends?

2. Of these three best friends, which friends do you feel gets the best grades in school assignments/work?

3. If you were to look at these three friends, which friend would you say would most likely become a doctor? A dog catcher? A

restaurant owner? What if the doctor was the person you chose for the dog catcher? What if the restaurant owner was the person you chose for the doctor?

Scenario 4-

James loves playing football. Playing football helps James to deal with the parts of his day that are hard to talk about and figure out. Anything related to football gives James a reason to smile about his rough moments. Yesterday, James found a dollar on the steps of the post office and bought four chocolate chip muffins from the market. When James returned home from playing football with four chocolate chip muffins and 60 cents, his brother Alan punched him in the stomach and took 2 muffins and the 60 cents from James. James heard Alan say to him that if he told their mother or stepfather about the muffins and the 60 cents he would do worse than punch him in the stomach once. James wept at his brother's words more than at the pain in his stomach.

1. What are three things that James can say to himself while throwing that football in the air and catching it that may ease his troubles?

2. Do you think that James knows that he is loved and needed?

3. Alan learned that his best friend had cancer on the morning that James found the dollar and bought the chocolate chip muffins. When he saw James with the chocolate chip muffins and the 60 cents, his response of punching James in the stomach and taking his muffins and change were reactions to the bad news that he learned about his best friend. What are two things that Alan could have done to deal with his bad news?

4.   What are two things that you would say to James if you were James' teacher? If you were Alan's classmate? If you were James and Alan's mother?

Activity 6- Goal Mapping

This idea of goal mapping is a process that can assist in creating functional steps towards achieving your goals. In goal mapping, one begins to determine the necessary steps that create a goal's realization. This activity will provide some instruction to help goal setting become a realistic part of our life. Goal mapping is the acknowledgement of a goal's working parts. Below you will find a goal mapping structure and you will take a few minutes to revisit the goals you listed in Activity #2. You got this!!!

Example-

Goal Number 1- <u>*I would like to get a library card*</u> *(1 month away)*

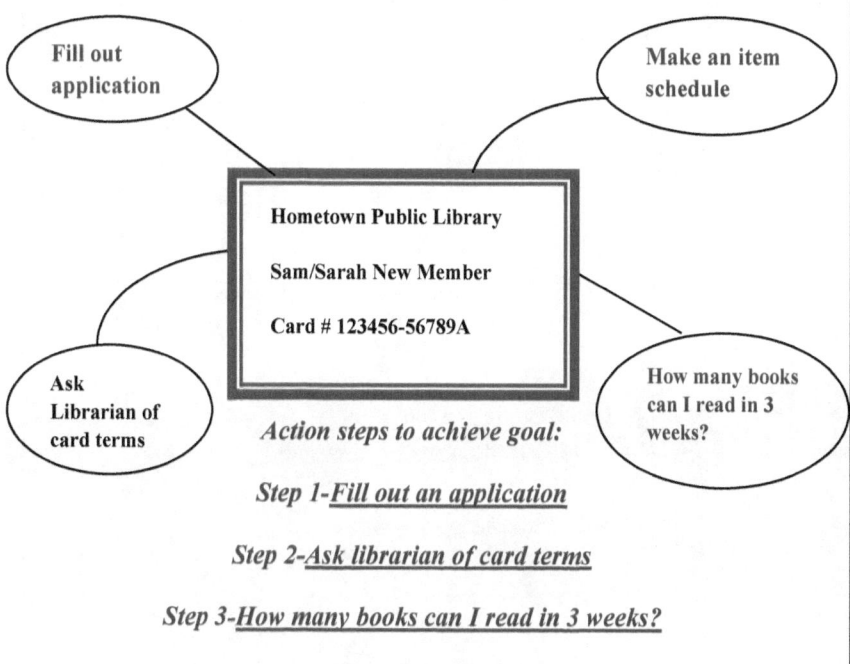

Fill out application

Make an item schedule

Hometown Public Library

Sam/Sarah New Member

Card # 123456-56789A

Ask Librarian of card terms

How many books can I read in 3 weeks?

Action steps to achieve goal:

Step 1-<u>*Fill out an application*</u>

Step 2-<u>*Ask librarian of card terms*</u>

Step 3-<u>*How many books can I read in 3 weeks?*</u>

Step 4-<u>*Make an item schedule.*</u>

Goal Number 2- _____(length of time from now)

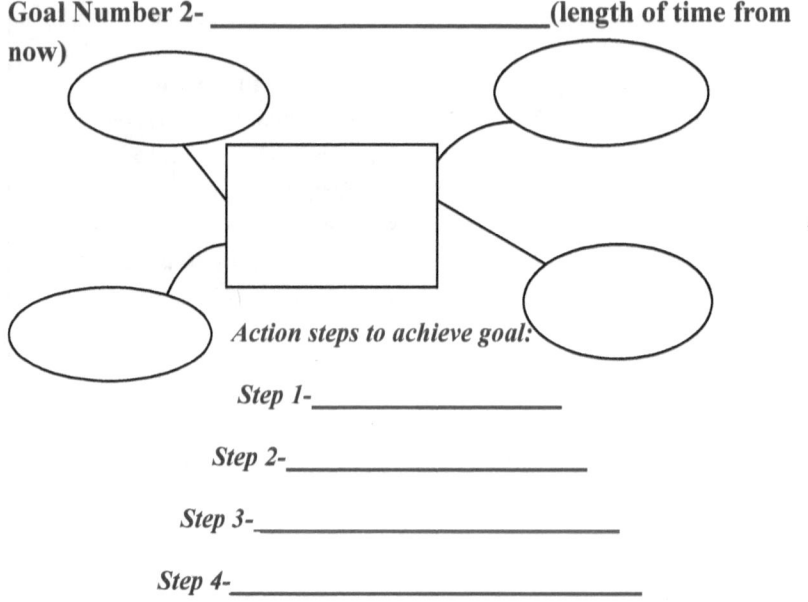

Action steps to achieve goal:

*Step 1-*_____

*Step 2-*_____

*Step 3-*_____

*Step 4-*_____

Goal Number 3- _____(length of time from now)

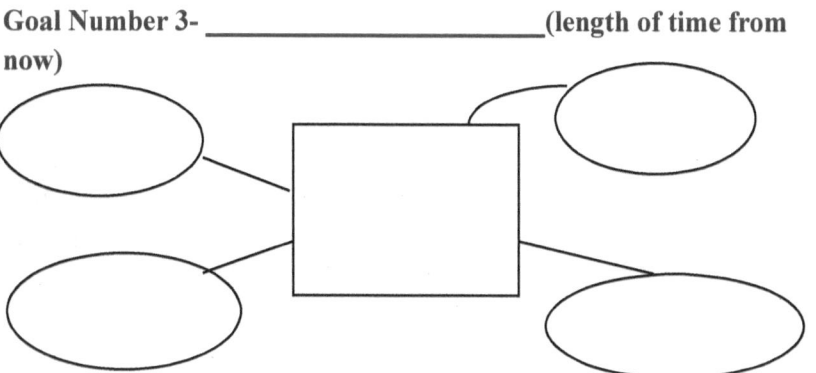

Action steps to achieve goal:

Step 1-_____

Step 2-_____

Step 3-_____

Step 4-_____